Breastfeeding
Your Premature Baby

By Gwen Gotsch

LA LECHE LEAGUE INTERNATIONAL
SCHAUMBURG, ILLINOIS

La Leche League International
1400 N. Meacham Road
Schaumburg, Illinois 60173-4840 USA
847-519-7730
www.lalecheleague.org

Photo Credits: Cover photo by John Roleson;
page 5, Gene Cranston Anderson; page 30,
© Mühlmann (Austria); page 36, Judy Torgus,
page 37, © Christa Herzog; page 39, Dale
Pfeiffer; page 43, David Wernick; page 50,
David Wernick; David Wernick; Elaine Caper;
page 53, Bill Skees

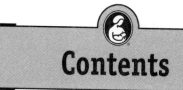

Contents

Chapter 1
Breastfeeding Basics

Human milk is the best food for human newborns, whether they're born healthy and full-term or early with problems. Human milk provides superior nutrition, protects against disease, and enhances infant development. This is why the American Academy of Pediatrics recommends breastfeeding as the standard for all infants. Anything else is second-best. Many mothers choose to breastfeed for these reasons—and because they want to experience the closeness that comes with nursing a baby.

Premature birth can make breastfeeding more challenging, but receiving human milk can be critical for these babies. How breast-feeding will be affected depends on a number of things: the baby's age and condition, the mother's health, the support and informa-tion available to her, and some practical considerations. Some babies, who are only a few weeks early, will breastfeed soon after birth with few problems. Other mothers may have to express their milk with a breast pump for several weeks—or even months—before their babies will be able to nurse at the breast. But even for these mothers and babies, breastfeeding is definitely possible—and important.

1

Why Human Milk Is Important for Premature Infants

Premature babies, especially the youngest and tiniest of them, face many challenges. Not yet ready for life outside their mother's womb, they have immature digestive systems. For these babies, human milk offers significant nutritional advantages. The protein in human milk is easier to digest and is better suited to the infant's needs. Fat is an important source of energy for growth in premies, and human milk contains an enzyme, lipase, which helps the baby digest the milk fat more efficiently. In the first weeks after birth, the milk of mothers of preterm babies contains greater amounts of protein, fat, sodium, iron, chloride, and other nutrients than milk from mothers of term infants. Although these differences start to disappear about one month after birth, some differences are evident for up to six months. The extra nutritional boost may help premies grow and develop.

Human milk's most impressive benefit for babies in neonatal nurseries is the way it protects from infection, and milk from mothers of preterm infants contains higher levels of many anti-infective factors. Immature immune systems have a more difficult time fighting off invaders, so the live cells and other immune factors in mother's milk are especially important to the premie. Components of human milk also stimulate the development of the baby's own immune system.

Full-term breastfed babies generally have fewer and less severe problems with colds, diarrhea, allergies, and ear infections. Preterm infants who receive human milk have fewer infections and are less likely to develop necrotizing enterocolitis, a serious bowel disease that affects premature babies. Researchers and physicians agree that immunologic protection is a very compelling reason for feeding premature babies with human milk. It makes sense— human milk was designed by nature for human babies.

Ongoing research shows that human milk contains an array of hormones and enzymes, including various growth factors. These help babies' digestive, immune, and nervous systems mature. Feedings of human milk are associated with better visual develop-

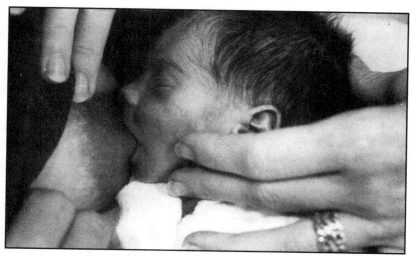

Breastfeeding your premature baby is something only you can do for him.

ment in premature infants and with significantly higher IQ scores later in childhood.

Breastfeeding is important to your premature baby's physical health and development, but it is also important to you and your feelings of attachment to your baby. Only the baby's mother—you—can provide human milk for him. Giving him your milk, even if he is not ready to nurse at the breast, creates a physical closeness between the two of you similar to your connection during pregnancy. Nurses and doctors may be the ones taking care of your baby from day to day, but you provide the milk that helps him grow and thrive. For many women, breastfeeding matters a great deal for this very reason.

Even if you're undecided about breastfeeding in the days following your baby's birth, it's a good idea to begin pumping milk for your baby. Your breasts are going to produce milk in the days after birth whether you decide to breastfeed or not—so you might as well give this milk to your baby. The early milk, called colostrum, contains very high levels of antibodies and other substances that protect against infection. Even a few feedings of human milk will benefit your baby. Also, it is much easier to bring in a good milk supply if you start pumping the first day or two after birth. Waiting a week and then deciding that you want to breastfeed makes it more difficult to establish milk production—although it can be done. If you decide later that you want to stop pumping, you can taper off gradually over several days and your breasts will stop making milk.

How Breastfeeding Works

Knowing how your body makes milk will help you understand the process of pumping milk for your baby and introducing your baby to the breast. It can also help you solve any problems that may arise.

In the first few days after birth, the breasts produce small amounts of the early milk called colostrum, which contains especially high levels of immunological factors. As hormone levels shift in the days following delivery, and the mother's estrogen and progesterone levels drop, the breasts begin to produce more milk. This is often referred to as the milk "coming in," and it can be very dramatic. Unless the milk is removed from the breasts by a nursing baby or with a pump, the mother's breasts may become painfully engorged.

The baby's nursing stimulates the brain to release two hormones: prolactin and oxytocin. Prolactin is the milk-making hormone. It tells the glands in the breast to make milk. Frequent removal of milk from the breasts by a nursing baby or by a pump keeps prolactin levels high, stimulating production of more milk.

Another hormone, oxytocin, causes cells around the glands to contract and squeeze the milk down into the milk sinuses, located behind the areola (the dark area around the nipple), where it is easily available to the baby as he nurses. This is called the milk ejection reflex or "let-down." Some mothers feel a tingling in their breasts when the milk lets down; others do not notice when the let-down occurs. If the baby is nursing, the mother will notice more frequent swallowing. If she's pumping, she will see an increased flow or spray of milk from her breasts into the pump when the let-down occurs. The let-down may occur even when the baby is not nursing, if, for example, the mother thinks about her baby or hears a baby crying.

At the beginning of the feeding the baby gets foremilk, which is stored in the milk sinuses behind the areola. The foremilk satisfies the baby's thirst. The let-down releases hindmilk, which is higher in fat than the foremilk. It's important that nursing or pumping sessions last long enough to trigger one or more let-downs, so that the baby will get the fat needed for growth.

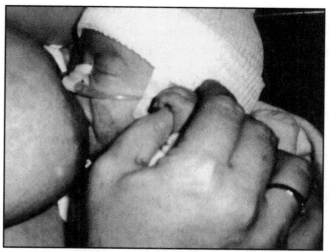

Pumping regularly means there will be a good supply of milk when your baby is ready to nurse.

Signals for continuing milk production

Once milk production begins, it works on the principle of supply and demand, or more accurately, demand and supply. When the baby breastfeeds and takes milk from the breast, the mother's body responds by making more milk. The more milk the baby takes and the more often the baby nurses, the more milk the mother's body makes. When the baby takes less milk, the mother's body slows down production. If no milk is removed from the breast, the breast gradually stops making milk. It takes a few days for the mother's body to make these adjustments between demand and supply, especially in the early weeks.

How breastfeeding works when the baby can't nurse. When a newborn baby is unable to nurse at the breast, the mother must remove milk from her breasts with a breast pump or hand expression in order to tell her body to continue to produce milk. Most mothers find that an electric breast pump is the most efficient and effective way to express their milk, but you can also use a manual pump or a technique called hand-expression. The milk can be refrigerated and given to the baby within the next 48 hours or it can be immediately frozen for later use. Expressing milk serves two purposes: it provides human milk for the baby's feedings and it signals the mother's body to keep producing milk, so that one day, when the baby is ready to nurse at the breast, there will be milk there.

When are premies ready to nurse at the breast?

Some premature babies who are older, bigger, and healthier will be able to nurse at the breast right away, or within a few days of birth. They may have a more difficult time learning to nurse than full-term babies, or they may feed for shorter time periods or more often. Very low birthweight babies are not able to breastfeed right away. They may be fed with special intravenous solutions at first. Later they may be given their mother's milk through a tube running from the nose or mouth to the stomach. This is called gavage or nasogastric feeding. When they are ready for nipple feedings, whether from bottle or breast, they may take some time learning to suck effectively and to coordinate sucking, breathing, and swallowing.

Breastfeeding a premature baby calls for extra effort, but it's worth it. As Jo-Anne Montgomery, the mother of Shannon, born nine weeks premature, wrote: "Nursing my baby daughter has been, and still is, one of the greatest pleasures of my life. Because we are a nursing couple, I am convinced that we were able to stay close and in tune with each other, even while Shannon was in the hospital."

Chapter 2
Expressing Your Milk

When a baby is unable to nurse at the breast, the mother must express her milk in order to maintain a milk supply. How soon the mother can begin to express depends on her condition and her situation, but generally, the earlier the better. Expressing milk eight to ten times a day in the first week to ten days after birth will help a mother establish a good milk supply.

Obtaining an Electric Pump

If hospital staff members have not discussed pumping your breasts with you, you will need to ask one of the nurses or the hospital's lactation consultant about obtaining and using a hospital-quality automatic electric breast pump. This is the most effective and most convenient way to express breast milk. Most hospitals have electric breast pumps available for mothers whose infants are unable to nurse at the breast. During the time that you are hospitalized, a pump should be available to you in your hospital room. There may also be a pump room near the neonatal intensive care nursery. After you are discharged from the hospital, you may need to rent or purchase a pump to use at home.

Hospital-quality automatic electric breast pumps are expensive to purchase, but they can be rented at reasonable rates on a weekly or monthly basis. Medical insurance should cover the cost if the baby's doctor writes specific orders saying the baby is premature and must have human milk. The doctor's letter could also point out that research has shown that an automatic electric pump is necessary to maintain a mother's milk supply. Hospital personnel can help you arrange to rent an electric breast pump to use at home; or you can contact the breast pump companies listed at the end of this book for more information about breast pump depots in your area. Your local La Leche League Leader can also assist you in locating a pump.

You will be given a collection kit to use with the electric breast pump. This includes a flange that fits over the breast, a collection bottle, and some tubing. You can set up the kit to pump both breasts at once; "double-pumping" takes less time and usually yields more milk. A nurse or lactation consultant can help you learn to use the pump; you can also consult the instruction book that comes with it.

An electric breast pump may look a little frightening at first—lots of pieces and tubes going everywhere. Keep in mind that the pump will help you give your precious milk to your baby. This will motivate you to master the mechanics.

Other Kinds of Breast Pumps

Hand-operated pumps and the smaller electric or battery-operated pumps are not as efficient and easy to use as automatic electric pumps and often are not adequate for establishing and maintaining a good milk supply. A mother whose baby is not yet nursing well at the breast usually needs an automatic electric pump to maintain her milk supply.

If you decide to purchase a smaller pump for occasional use or to carry with you, be sure to explore all your options. Breast pumps can be purchased in drug stores, stores that sell baby equipment, or from some La Leche League Leaders and lactation consultants. The collection kit that comes with an electric pump may

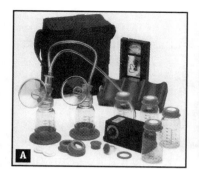
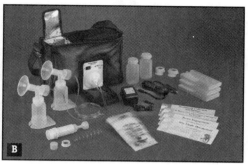

*Samples of electric, battery, and manual pumps a mother may want to purchase:
(A) Nurture III Double Electric Breastpump; (B) Medela Pump in Style;*

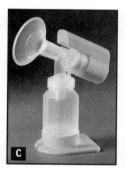
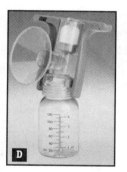
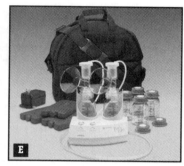

*(C) Medela Mini Electric Pump; (D) Ameda Egnell One Handed Pump;
(E) Ameda Egnell Purely Yours Pump*

include attachments that enable you to use the equipment as a manual pump. Besides hand-operated pumps, there are also some lower-priced electric or battery-operated pumps on the market. The companies that make high quality automatic electric pumps (the kind you rent) also manufacture less expensive electric pumps that can be purchased through rental depots. These may be a better choice than the pump on the shelf at the drug store.

The simplest type of manual pump creates suction using a rubber bulb and looks like a bicycle horn. It cannot be adequately sterilized, and the suction cannot be controlled. This kind of pump should not be used to pump milk for a premature baby.

How to Pump

1. Have your equipment clean, ready, and assembled. Get a glass of water or juice. Wash your hands.

2. Sit down and take a moment to relax. Think pleasant thoughts. Imagine yourself in a favorite place, on a beach, near a stream. Or think loving thoughts about your baby. A picture of the baby or a blanket used by the baby that smells like him may help you. Imagine the feel of his skin, or the soft hair on his head.

3. Many mothers find that breast massage helps them to relax and stimulates the let-down reflex. Start the massage in the outer area of the breast, near the armpit. Use the tips of your fingers to make several circular motions in the same spot. Then move your fingers to the next area, moving around the breast in a spiral, working toward the nipple area.

4. Center your nipple in the flange of the pump. If the pump has different size flanges, use the one that fits the best; it should surround the areola without being too big. The flange should form a tight seal around the areola. Moistening it with warm water may help improve the seal.

5. If you are using an electric pump, turn it on at the lowest setting. If you are using a manual pump, operate it gently. As you pump, you may want to increase the suction, but not to the point where it's uncomfortable. You need to use enough suction to be effective, but not so much that your nipples get sore. You will see the nipple and areola moving back and forth inside the flange. When the let-down reflex is activated, you will see sprays or streams of milk

6. Pump until the spray of milk slows down or stops, then pump a minute or two more, in case the milk flow resumes. The last few drops of milk you pump have the highest fat content, and fat provides the calories your baby needs to grow. If you are pumping both breasts at the same time, you will probably pump for about fifteen minutes per session once your milk has "come in."

7. If you are pumping each breast separately, switch to the other side when the milk flow slows or stops. Pump the second breast until the milk flow slows, and then return to the first breast and pump for another five minutes, or until the milk stops. Repeat for another five minutes on the second breast. If the milk is flowing well, you may want to pump each breast a third time.

8. Carefully transfer the milk from the collecting bottle to the storage container, label it with your baby's name and the date and time, and refrigerate it. Be careful not to touch the inside of either container or to let the milk touch your fingers. Store your milk in feeding-sized portions. Your baby's nurse can suggest how much milk you should put in a single container.

9. Use cold water to rinse the parts of the pump that come in contact with milk. Then wash these parts of the pump in hot soapy water and rinse thoroughly. Some pump parts can be washed in the dishwasher.

Hand-Expression

Hand-expression is a handy skill to have in case you're caught somewhere without your pump and your breasts are beginning to feel uncomfortably full. It requires minimal equipment—only a container in which to collect the milk. If you are hand-expressing only to relieve fullness, you can lean over a sink or express the milk into a towel.

To hand-express milk, position the thumb above the breast and the fingers below, about 1 to 1½ inches (2½-4 cm) behind the nipple. Push the thumb and fingers straight back into the chest wall, then roll them forward to compress the milk sinuses underneath the skin. Be careful not to slide the fingers along the skin; this can cause skin burns. Work on one area until the milk flow stops, then rotate the hand around the breast and repeat the process to reach all the milk ducts. Express for five minutes on one side, five minutes on the other, then repeat. (For more detailed information on hand-expression and breast massage, see THE WOMANLY ART OF BREASTFEEDING.)

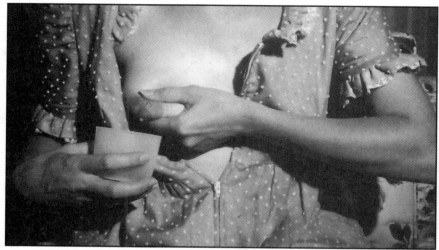

Hand-expression is a skill you may find useful.

When to Express Milk

Milk expression should imitate how often a baby nurses, and new-borns nurse eight to twelve times a day. Frequent pumping—every two to three hours—will help you establish a good milk supply in the first weeks after birth when your body is primed by pregnancy and childbirth to make milk. This can be important for later milk production. You may pump more milk than your baby needs, but this can be an advantage in the weeks to come. Even if your milk supply decreases as the weeks go by, if you start with a lot of milk, you will still have a good supply of milk when it is time for your baby to begin feedings at the breast.

If you must pump for many weeks you may eventually find that you don't need to pump as frequently. One study found that mothers needed a minimum of five pumping sessions each day, for a total of 100 minutes, to maintain a milk supply while the baby was not nursing. If you find your milk supply decreasing, be sure to pump more often.

Frequent pumping is more effective than longer pumping sessions spaced at wider intervals. Some mothers wake at night or in the early morning to pump, especially if their breasts are feeling uncomfortably full. Others find that uninterrupted sleep helps both their milk supply and their ability to cope with the daily pressures that go along with having a hospitalized baby. When your baby is ready to begin nursing at the breast, you may want to increase the number of pumping sessions each day to build up your milk supply. You might also want to pump more frequently when you know that your baby will soon be coming home from the hospital.

If you have questions about expressing milk or the breast pump itself, talk to a La Leche League Leader, a nurse who is knowledgeable about breastfeeding, or a lactation consultant, if one is available in your hospital. The instructions that come with the pump can answer many of your questions about operating it and cleaning it. While you are still hospitalized, hospital personnel will help you with cleaning and sterilizing. When you return home, this can be a way in which the baby's father or other support person helps out. Having more than one collection kit to use with an electric pump cuts down on the time needed to sterilize equipment.

Storing Expressed Milk

Expressed human milk does not look like cow's milk from a carton. It is thin and bluish-looking; as it stands in the refrigerator, the cream rises to the top. Human milk, like any other fresh food, is perishable. It must be handled carefully, stored in the refrigerator or freezer, and used promptly. When human milk is given to premature or sick infants, careful handling is especially important.

Milk that will be given to your premature baby within 48 hours after expressing can be stored in the refrigerator. Milk that will be kept for a longer period of time must be frozen immediately. Freezing destroys some, though by no means all, of breast milk's immunologic factors, so whenever possible, it is better for your baby to receive fresh milk. However, in the early days your baby may not be ready for milk feedings, and you may find that you have an ample milk supply in the first days after your milk comes in. Pumping and freezing the colostrum, as well as the early milk, will provide your baby with valuable immunities when he is ready for milk feedings. Some mothers find that their milk supply decreases after several weeks of pumping; having milk stored in the freezer can be reassuring when a growing baby begins to take more milk each day.

Transporting milk to the hospital. You must take care that milk does not warm or thaw when transporting it to the hospital. Pack it tightly in a small ice chest or insulated container, and use a folded towel to fill any empty space. You can bring your milk to the hospital each day when you visit your baby. If you live far away from the hospital or cannot visit regularly for some other reason, you may be able to arrange for family, friends, or even a hospital employee who lives nearby to transport your milk.

Freezing your milk. Milk expressed for premature or sick infants should be stored in sterile, airtight containers. Like water, milk expands when it freezes, so leave about an inch of space at the top. Each container should be labeled with your name, your baby's name, the date and time of expression, and any medications you are currently taking. (The hospital may be able to provide you with labels preprinted with your baby's name and identification number.) The nursery nurses will want to use the oldest milk first, and clear, easy-to-read labels will make their job easier. Freeze milk in feeding-size portions to avoid wasting milk. Check with your baby's nurses for the amount of milk to put in each container.

Place your milk in the back of the freezer compartment of your refrigerator, away from the door and in a frost-free refrigerator, away from the defrosting fan. If possible, store your milk in a deep freeze where the temperature stays below 0 degrees Fahrenheit (-19 degrees Centigrade). Frozen milk should be given to premature babies within three months of expression.

Storage containers. Expressed milk is usually stored in a hard-sided container made of plastic or glass or in some kind of plastic bag. Each kind of storage container has advantages and disadvantages. Plastic bags take up less room, and some types can even be attached directly to the pump to collect the milk. However, hard-sided containers do a better job protecting the milk. Some of the immunities in milk, as well as some of the fat and vitamins, may cling to the sides of plastic bags. Plastic bags may be difficult to seal, and the bags may burst during freezing or leak when the milk is thawed.

Freezer milk bags specifically designed to store frozen human milk may be available from pump rental agents. (They can also be ordered from LLLI. See Resources.) These bags are preferable to the thinner, disposable plastic bags used in bottle-feeding systems. If you store your milk in plastic bags, leave some room at the top for the milk to expand as it freezes (otherwise the bag may burst) and fasten the top securely. Use a twist-tie if the bag does not come with a clip or a seal. Double-bagging protects against breakage when you use the thinner bags. Place the bags of milk inside another container to support and protect them in the freezer.

It may be difficult for nurses to remove thawed milk from a plastic bag without accidentally touching the milk. One way to avoid contamination is to snip off the bottom corner of the bag with a sterile scissors and pour the milk out. Some milk storage bags have built-in pour spouts.

Hospitals often provide milk storage containers for mothers who are pumping milk for their babies. Ask about these. The bill for your baby's care probably contains a "feeding fee," which to be fair, should cover some kind of container for the valuable milk that you are providing free of charge.

Your baby's doctors and nurses may have other specific suggestions for you about handling, storing, and transporting your milk. Ask them about their preferences.

How Your Milk Will Be Given to Your Baby

Your baby's first milk feedings will probably be gavage feedings; your milk will be slowly pushed through a tube that leads from the baby's nose into the stomach, or the milk will be allowed to run into the baby's stomach by force of gravity. If colostrum is available—fresh or frozen—it should be the first food your baby receives.

It is often possible for premature babies to receive fresh milk (refrigerated rather than frozen) for all or almost all of their feedings, especially when the baby is very small. If you pump at the hospital when you visit the baby, you can ask that this milk be given to your baby immediately—without ever being refrigerated. This will maximize the benefits of giving your baby your milk.

Commercial fortifiers are often added to human milk when it is given to premature babies, especially very low birthweight infants. The fortifier provides additional protein and minerals to meet the unique nutritional needs of premies. If your baby's caretakers are adding nutrients to your milk before giving it to your baby, don't feel that this means your milk is inadequate or not good enough for your baby. Your milk is the foundation of good nutrition for your baby, and it also provides valuable protection against infection, which cannot be duplicated by special premie formulas or fortifiers. When your baby gets bigger, breastfeeding can be his only source of nourishment until he is ready for solid foods.

Some researchers are experimenting with fortifying human milk with the mother's own hindmilk. By increasing the fat content of the milk, they increase the calories available for growth. You can increase the fat content of the milk you pump by pumping longer, until your breasts seem empty. If the doctors are concerned about your baby's growth, you might ask if they would try giving your baby mainly the milk expressed later in pumping sessions, after you've experienced a let-down. You will need to switch collection bottles during pumping to make this possible.

Chapter 3
Problems with Pumping

Pumping—the equipment, the instructions, the containers, and the schedules—may seem confusing or overwhelming at first. If you are pumping on the first day or two after the birth, before your milk "comes in," you won't see much colostrum in the container (although these small amounts are very valuable!). In a few days, you'll be more familiar with the pump, your milk will become plentiful, and you'll develop a routine. Pumping is a learned skill, as is breastfeeding a baby, and you may feel awkward while you're learning.

The Let-Down Reflex

Pumping does not trigger the let-down reflex as effectively as a nursing baby, and without a let-down, you will not be able to pump much milk. It may be difficult sometimes to relax and allow the let-down or milk-ejection reflex to operate. Here are some suggestions:

- Follow a set routine when you pump. Pump in the same place, in a comfortable chair that supports your arms in a comfortable position.

- Minimize distractions. Turn off the phone, play some relaxing music. Have everything ready that you will need, including a glass of juice or water, a nutritious snack, and maybe something to read.

- A warm shower or warm moist washcloths applied to the breasts can help you relax and stimulate the let-down before you begin pumping. You can massage your breasts in the shower. (You may not want to do this before every pumping session, but it can really help if you've been rushing around or are especially tense.)

- Get away from it all in your mind. Picture yourself in a pleasant place—on a warm sandy beach, with the waves lapping at the shore; near a mountain stream, somewhere enjoying a tropical breeze.

- Think about your baby. Look at a picture, or imagine your baby cuddled against your breast. Some mothers call the nursery just before pumping to find out how the baby is doing. It may be possible to pump right at the hospital when you are visiting your baby, even while sitting next to the crib. If your baby is getting tube feedings, ask that the fresh milk be given to him right away.

- Thoughts about your baby, hearing a baby cry, or sometimes other events can stimulate the let-down reflex. If you feel your milk let down or notice leaking between pumping sessions, take advantage of it. Pump for a few minutes.

- Specific mental images can help your milk flow. Imagine a waterfall or a fountain of milk—or whatever works for you.

- If you have older children who want your attention while you're pumping, plan ahead for their needs. Set up your pump next to the couch so your toddler or preschooler can sit next to you. Read books together or have quiet activities ready that you can share.

Pumping five to eight times a day (or more) will seem tedious at times. Many mothers say they feel more attached to the pump than to their baby. Keep in mind that you and your milk are very important to your baby. Seek out some support—someone who will listen to your fears and worries and complaints. Call a supportive friend, perhaps another breastfeeding mother, or a La Leche League Leader. Talk to someone who knows that while breastfeeding is important to mothers and babies, it does have its ups and downs, and in some situations, can be very challenging. Even if this person herself has not been in your exact situation, she can sympathize with you and understand your frustrations.

Keeping Up Your Milk Supply

Many mothers find that the amount of milk they can pump begins to decrease after several weeks. This is normal (a pump does not stimulate milk production as efficiently as a nursing baby), but it can be upsetting, especially if the baby's appetite is increasing at the same time your milk supply is dwindling. How much milk you produce may also vary depending on your baby's condition.

It's natural to focus your attention on how much milk you're producing from one pumping session to the next. But try not to worry; focus on long-term goals instead—perhaps providing milk when your baby is ready for tube feedings or having milk in your breasts when your baby is ready to begin breastfeeding. Here are some things you can do to increase your milk supply while pumping:

• Pump more frequently. If you are pumping five times a day, try to pump seven or eight times a day until you see an increase in your milk supply. Once your milk supply increases, you can probably return to your previous pumping schedule and still maintain the increased milk production. One study found that mothers needed to pump at least five times per day for a total of 100 minutes of pumping in order to keep up a milk supply. This may be enough for some mothers, not enough for others.

• Frequent pumping is especially important in the first weeks postpartum to establish a good milk supply. Young full-term babies nurse every two to three hours, and pumping should imitate the behavior of a breastfed baby.

- Frequent shorter pumping sessions are better than longer ones spaced farther apart.

- Follow a regular pumping routine. Take time to relax and massage your breasts before you pump. Look at a picture of your baby.

- Pump at the hospital before and after you visit your baby. Bring the pump to your baby's bedside and pump there.

- Ask your baby's caregivers about kangaroo care. This involves holding your baby out of the isolette skin-to-skin against your breasts. The physical closeness is good for babies and skin-to-skin contact often helps boost a mother's milk supply. (See Chapter 4 for more details about kangaroo care.)

- Get more rest. Take a nap during the day. Get to bed early. Pump in the middle of the night if you awaken, but don't lose sleep over pumping.

- Take care of yourself. Concentrate your energies on things that are really important—visits with your baby in the hospital, time with your spouse, caring for your other children, resting, pumping. You are recovering from pregnancy and childbirth and dealing with intense stress. Your body and mind need special care.

- Get help with household tasks, errands, child care. When friends offer to help, be ready with specific assignments. Don't think you have to do everything yourself.

- Eat well. Although even undernourished mothers can produce good quality milk, you need to pay attention to what you're eating to stay healthy during this stressful period. This is not a time to skip meals or try to lose weight. Bring healthy snacks and juices with you to the hospital. Cheese, fresh fruit, whole-grain breads, raw vegetables, nuts, yogurt, and granola are easy to grab from the refrigerator or cupboard as you head out the door. Carry a thermos of water or juice so you won't be tempted to quench your thirst with soft drinks or coffee. Have a glass of water or juice every time you sit down to pump.

Milk supplies often fluctuate with the baby's condition. When you are very worried about the baby's health, you may not be able to pump much milk. This is normal, part of the complex emotions involved in having a baby who is very ill. Keep pumping, so that you will have some milk in your breasts when your baby is ready for feedings at the breast. You can increase your milk supply with more frequent pumping as the baby's condition improves.

Sore Nipples

Pumping sometimes leads to sore nipples. Here are some suggestions to heal sore nipples and prevent them from reoccurring.

- Check the directions to be sure you are using the pump correctly.

- Try pumping more frequently but for shorter periods of time. Pump on the least sore side first.

- Use breast massage to get the let-down reflex started before you pump; the sore feeling often lessens as the milk starts to flow.

- Try using the larger flange on the pump. Be sure the nipple is centered so that it doesn't rub against the side of the flange.

- Use the least amount of suction needed to maintain the milk flow.

- After feedings, express a little milk onto the nipple. This can aid healing.

- Cracked or sore nipples heal best when the skin retains its internal moisture. To prevent nipple skin from drying out, after pumping pat your nipples dry and soften a pea-sized portion of Lansinoh for Breastfeeding Mothers® between clean fingertips. Apply to each nipple. Gently pat it on, don't rub it in. Lansinoh is the purest and safest brand of USP modified lanolin and does not have to be removed before feeding the baby or pumping your milk. It prevents scabs from forming on any cracks, eases pain, and hastens healing. (See Resources.)

Flat or inverted nipples. If you have flat or inverted nipples, you may find that pumping helps them to protrude. You can tell if your nipples are flat or inverted by squeezing gently at the base of the nipple. If the nipple shrinks back into the breast or barely protrudes, the baby may have a difficult time grasping the nipple to nurse. To stretch the nipple and help it protrude, try rolling the nipple gently between your fingers several times before pumping.

Reducing Bacteria Levels in Pumped Milk

Breast milk is not sterile. The same types of bacteria normally found on the skin of the nipple and areola are also present in expressed milk. Human milk contains a number of antibacterial factors, which help to keep bacterial growth to a minimum when milk is stored. However, because premies are more vulnerable to infection than full-term infants, you must be very careful in handling and storing the milk so that bacteria remain at minimal levels. The Neonatal Intensive Care Unit (NICU) where your baby is being cared for may have specific instructions for you to follow.

Some neonatal nurseries regularly check the bacteria levels in pumped milk, while others do not find this necessary. Bacteria in the milk will not harm a healthy full-term or a larger premature baby, but there is some concern that higher levels of bacteria in milk could make a very tiny baby ill. Decisions about acceptable bacteria levels in expressed milk are best made on a case-by-case basis.

If your baby's caregivers are concerned about bacteria in your milk, there are several things you can do to bring down the levels.

- Be very careful with your handling of pumping and milk storage equipment. Follow the manufacturer's instructions on cleaning or sterilizing the pump and the containers.

- Wash your hands thoroughly before pumping, and clean under your nails.

- Avoid touching the inside of milk containers and the inside of the pump flange that fits over your nipple.

- Some nurseries may suggest discarding the first 10 cc (about two teaspoons) of milk you pump to lower bacteria counts, but this has not been shown to be effective. It can be very discouraging to throw away milk, especially if you are able to pump only small amounts at a time.

- Another alternative, cleansing the nipple and areola area with an antibacterial soap before pumping, is probably also unnecessary. Normal everyday hygiene and careful handwashing should be adequate to keep bacteria levels in your milk within safe limits.

If the doctors and nurses caring for your baby are concerned about bacteria levels in your expressed milk, you may have to follow a more elaborate pumping routine until your baby is bigger, older, or healthier.

Medications and Human Milk

Most medications are compatible with breastfeeding full-term babies, and most medications are also compatible with pumping milk for a premature or ill newborn. However, some medications taken by the mother can cause problems for babies, and premature infants are more sensitive to the effects of drugs than full-term babies. If you are taking any prescription drugs, using any over-the-counter medications, or other substances, you should share this information with your baby's doctors and indicate this on the labels of the milk you pump. It may be necessary for you to discard the milk you pump while taking certain medications. This can be very discouraging—but continuing the frequent pumping, even if the milk is not given to your baby, is important to maintaining your milk supply for the days when either you are no longer using the medication or your baby is more mature and the drug is no longer a problem.

If your baby's doctors have questions about medications in human milk, encourage them to seek information from specialists beyond the local hospital or the drug's manufacturer, whose principal concern is avoiding liability. A computer search may yield more information about a specific drug. (See References at the end of this book.) Your local La Leche League Leader can direct you to a resource person who may be able to provide further information. There are many factors to consider when making decisions about medications in mother's milk, and the risks of giving a baby artificial formula should be considered along with the risks of the drug.

Getting Help with Problems

If you're feeling discouraged about pumping and breastfeeding or if you need some help with a breastfeeding problem, talk to a La Leche League Leader or someone at the hospital who is knowledgeable about breastfeeding. You need support. Family and friends may not understand why you go to the trouble to pump your milk, and they may—with the best of intentions—suggest quitting as the obvious solution to any difficulties that you're having. Talk to someone who understands both the importance of pumping milk for your baby and the challenges you face. Problems can be solved with the help and encouragement of someone who believes in what you are doing.

Chapter 4
Parenting a Premie

Even when the baby is doing well, the whole experience of premature labor and delivery can be overwhelming. At a time when you may still have been planning your baby's nursery or just starting childbirth classes, you're confronted with medical terms, technology, and decisions you never even anticipated. When a baby is critically ill, the experience is that much more intense.

Still, you are this baby's parent. You are the one who is ultimately responsible for her, though you may not feel like there is much you can do for her in the hospital. But take the time to get to know her, to spend time with her, so that you can begin to feel like her mother.

Your Feelings and Worries

It's normal to be confused and anxious, scared and worried when your baby is ill. It can be hard to concentrate with all these feelings churning away inside you. You may need to have medical information repeated for you. You may find yourself going back and retelling the circumstances of your baby's birth over and over again. You may feel angry or sad or disoriented—or all of these things at once. If your baby experiences repeated health crises, each new problem may force you to work through all of your emotions yet again.

Husbands and wives may be at different stages of dealing with their feelings, and each may feel very alone at times. It's important to take time to listen to each other during this stressful period.

Guilt can be a big problem for mothers when a baby is premature, critically ill, or experiencing developmental problems. Mothers, and fathers too, want to protect their children, to fix what's wrong, to make everything better. But realistically, many, many things in life are beyond our ability to control. Even when one is trying to do everything "right," things can go wrong. Medical problems can complicate breastfeeding. The many details of living can get in the way of spending time at your baby's crib. One lesson to be learned from difficult situations is that you do the best you can, and let go of the rest. Focus on what's most important, one day at a time, and what's possible. Don't be too hard on yourself.

Ask the nurses if there is a support group for parents of babies in the premature nursery or if there is another way for you to be in contact with parents who have been through a similar experience. Talking with other families who have experienced what you are going through can be very reassuring. These are people who can understand and accept your feelings, both positive and negative. A support group can also be a source of practical help in the days ahead. Experienced parents know many things you will need to know about your baby's care and development.

If your baby dies

Despite the best efforts of modern medicine, some babies are too tiny or have too many problems to survive. It may surprise you that your body continues to produce milk, even if your baby has died. You may experience uncomfortable engorgement which could develop into a breast infection if left untreated. Your doctor may suggest medication to suppress milk production, but medication may have side effects and is not always effective in ending lactation. An alternative is to express or pump only a little milk, just enough to relieve the discomfort, several times a day. You'll need to do this less often as your body gradually stops producing milk. You may also find it helpful to wear a firm bra for comfort and support, although binding the breasts tightly is not recommended as a way of suppressing lactation. Some mothers find it comforting to donate their expressed milk to a donor milk bank where it can be used for other sick or premature infants. (See Resources.)

The loss of a child is a devastating experience. It can help to share your grief with others who have faced a similar loss. There are several support groups for parents who have lost a child. You may want to get in touch with one of these groups so you can talk about your experience and share your feelings with others. The nursery staff or hospital social worker can put you in touch with a group near you.

Working with Health Professionals

The technology and terminology of the intensive care nursery can be frightening and intimidating. Talking to the doctors and nurses can help you get a better idea of what's going on with your baby. Write down your concerns and questions as they occur to you, so that you will remember them when you talk with your baby's caregivers. Make an effort to communicate regularly with your baby's caregivers. Find out when your baby's doctor is scheduled to be in the NICU so that you can talk to him or her in person as questions come up. Also ask the doctor how you can reach him or her at other times, and when is the best time to talk. Be polite, helpful, respectful—and honest about your concerns and wishes. You want the doctors and nurses to see you as an important member of the team caring for your baby.

You may find that there are one or two professionals who are particularly good at explaining things and at listening and responding to your concerns. Seek out those people, arrange to visit the nursery while they are working, and share your good moments as well as your worries with them. (They sometimes need a boost too.) The NICU may have a social worker who can assist you with non-medical issues. There may also be books and pamphlets available for parents, explaining medical procedures and other issues. The Resources listed in the back of this book can also help answer questions you may have.

Once your baby is past the critical stage, you may see less of the doctors and more of the nurses. Nurses, especially, can help you to see your baby as a tiny human being with special needs, more than just an extension of all the machinery. Medical professionals are becoming increasingly supportive of parents' need to form an attachment to their premature babies while they are in the hospital.

Sharing breastfeeding information with health professionals

Not all doctors and nurses working in neonatal intensive care units are knowledgeable about breastfeeding and human milk. There are tremendous differences between hospitals when it comes to policies and practices regarding breast milk and breastfeeding. The suggestions in this book are based on solid medical research and the advice of experienced neonatal care providers who are committed to giving premature infants their own mother's milk.

Some of what you read here may be new to the doctors and nurses caring for your baby—or different from the way they usually do things. You may have to assert yourself, tactfully but firmly, to be sure that your baby is getting your pumped milk, is getting fresh milk when it's available, has opportunities for skin-to-skin contact with you, or is allowed to begin nursing at the breast as soon as possible. Remind your baby's caregivers that breastfeeding is important to you and your baby. Let them know what you are willing to do to give your baby your milk.

One strategy that may be helpful, when you're told that one thing or another can't be done, is to ask "Is this your general policy, or is this advice specifically for my baby?" You don't need to change the unit's policy—only have it individualized for your baby. Decisions about kangaroo care (explained in the next chapter), about when a baby is allowed to nurse at the breast, and other issues should be based on your baby's condition—not broad policies. Share the information in this book, along with the reference list at the back with your baby's caregivers. Ask them to look up the reference material in their medical library or on the Internet if they have further questions about a specific issue.

Being in conflict with a health care provider is hard. A physician calls on tremendous amounts of highly specialized knowledge—knowledge that you and your baby depend on. You must be tactful and calm when expressing your preferences and listening to the doctor's advice. You must be willing to take responsibility as part of the team that is caring for your baby. You may need to make some compromises to arrive at a plan agreeable to everyone. Remember that all of you share the same goal—doing the best you can for your baby.

Getting to Know Your Baby

Spend as much time with your baby as you can. If the hospital is a long distance from your home, see if there is somewhere you can stay near the hospital—with friends or family or in a hotel. The hospital may be able to help you make arrangements so that you don't have to travel long distances or incur great expense to be near your baby. If you have other children at home, you'll need to balance their needs with those of your new baby. Seek out the support of friends and family. If people offer to help, be ready to suggest specific tasks they can do for you that will allow you to spend more time with your baby.

When you visit your baby in the neonatal nursery, plan on staying for a while. Ask for a comfortable chair so that you can sit beside your baby's isolette. You may be able to help with her care, or look into her eyes and touch and stroke her tiny body. She will know that somebody loves her, and this is very important. Be aware that some premies are very sensitive to stimulation, so watch your baby's signals to discover what kinds of sounds and touches are soothing and what kind may be overstimulating.

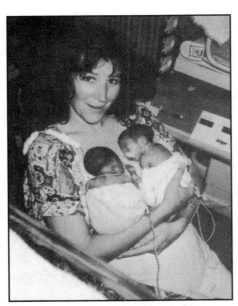

Kangaroo care provides measurable health benefits for premature babies.

Kangaroo care

Gentle, calming human touch actually produces health benefits for premature babies. Ongoing research into a practice called kangaroo care is showing that premies sleep better, breathe better, and stay warmer while held skin-to-skin in an upright position by a parent. This physical closeness also improves mothers' milk supplies.

The concept of kangaroo care began in a hospital in Bogota, Colombia that did not have enough incubators and other equipment to care for all the low birthweight babies. Mortality rates from infection and respiratory problems were high, and many of these impoverished mothers eventually abandoned newborn infants who were ill. Two neonatologists thought that perhaps mothers could care for their premies more effectively than the hospital, with its limited technological resources. So they asked mothers to "wear" their premature babies, tucked between their breasts, 24 hours a day. The experiment worked: mortality rates dropped, and mothers who used kangaroo care were much less likely to abandon their babies.

Since then, hospitals in Europe and North America have begun to adapt kangaroo care for use in intensive care nurseries by giving mothers and fathers the opportunity to hold their premature babies skin-to-skin. Babies who are in stable condition can be taken out of the isolette and held in a vertical position cradled against the mother's breasts or the father's bare chest. The baby is clothed in only a diaper and, perhaps, a warm cap, and parent and baby are covered with a receiving blanket. The parent reclines in a comfortable chair, and parent and baby stay together for an hour or more, while nurses monitor the baby's condition at regular intervals.

Kangaroo care gives parents of premature infants a great deal of emotional satisfaction. But the amazing feature of kangaroo care is the measurable health benefits for babies. Their breathing patterns and heart rates become more regular. They become less irritable. They may gaze quietly at a parent's face and then fall into a deep, restful, much-needed sleep. Studies have shown that the skin temperature of a mother's breast actually changes in response to her baby's need for warmth; even premature infants who otherwise need help in maintaining their body temperature do not get cold in kangaroo care.

Skin-to-skin contact with mother also helps to set the stage for nursing at the breast. If you express a few drops of milk onto your nipple (or if you experience a milk let-down), the baby can lick and nuzzle and smell and begin to learn where her nourishment comes from. Some nurses may even be willing to administer gavage feedings while your baby is cuddled at your breast. The physical contact with the baby is also important for mothers. It helps to increase your milk supply, improve your let-down, and remind you of your importance to your baby. (Have a towel or breast pad handy during kangaroo care, to absorb any milk that leaks from your breasts.)

You may want to pump your breasts before holding your baby skin-to-skin, so that her first attempts at sucking yield only a few drops of milk. She may not yet be ready to coordinate sucking, swallowing, and breathing. Be sure to pump your breasts again at the hospital when you are finished holding your baby. This physical closeness often enables mothers to pump significantly more milk.

Talk to the doctors and nurses about kangaroo care and share with them the references at the end of this book. Even if your baby is still on a respirator, you may be able to hold her while nurses monitor her reaction. Fathers can use kangaroo care, too; it helps them feel attached to their tiny infants.

If you would like to know more about kangaroo care or would like to be able to share more information about this concept with your baby's caregivers, read *Kangaroo Care: The Best You Can Do to Help Your Preterm Infant* by Susan M. Ludington-Hoe (available in bookstores and from LLLI). This book describes research on kangaroo care, tells when babies are ready to try it, gives detailed instructions, and also provides a guide to understanding your premie's behavior.

Chapter 5
Beginning to Breastfeed

Making the transition from pumping and tube feeding to nursing at the breast can be the most challenging part of breastfeeding a premature baby. It takes commitment, but the rewards are worth the effort.

This chapter presents detailed information about how babies latch on to the breast and suck effectively. Don't feel that you have to master all this information before putting your baby to the breast. Instead, use the various lists to fine-tune your breastfeeding as you and the baby become more experienced.

When to Begin

Some physicians feel that a premature baby should reach a certain age or weight before being allowed to breastfeed, or that the baby must first learn to suck from a bottle. However, research has shown that these are not valid criteria for determining if a baby is ready for breastfeeding and that babies may be ready to breastfeed earlier than some health care providers recognize.

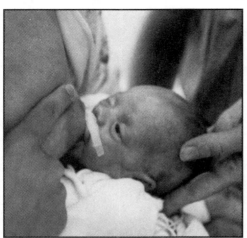

*A helper may need to provide support
behind the baby's head.*

More important factors for determining when a baby may nurse at the breast include the baby's overall condition, how well he tolerates milk fed by tube, and his ability to coordinate sucking, breathing, and swallowing. In some studies, premature infants as young as thirty-two weeks gestational age, weighing as little as 1100 grams, have been observed to nurse at the breast. Most pre-term infants will not nurse effectively until they are a little older or larger than this.

Pre-term infants may be ready to breastfeed well before they are ready to bottle-feed. Breastfeedings are less stressful than bottle-feedings. Sucking, swallowing, and breathing are more easily coordinated at the breast, and infants have more control over the milk flow. Also, introducing a baby to the breast before he is started on bottle-feedings makes it easier for him to learn to nurse.

Talk to your baby's care providers about when he will be ready to start nursing at the breast. You may want to share some of the references at the end of this book with them. Most physicians will want a nurse to monitor a baby closely during early feedings at the breast. They may also want to use the test-weighing technique described below to measure the amount of milk the baby receives.

Your Baby's First Feedings at the Breast

Early feedings will take time and patience. This is a learning process for both of you, and you may feel awkward and frustrated at times. It will probably take several breastfeeding sessions before your baby latches on and nurses well. Be patient, enjoy the cuddling and closeness (this is part of learning to breastfeed, too), and keep trying. These early feedings are the hardest part; breastfeeding will get easier.

Here are some suggestions to help you prepare for your baby's first feeding at the breast.

- Privacy and quiet are helpful. Your hospital may have a separate room where you can breastfeed, or you can ask for a screen or curtains.

- You'll need a chair with armrests, along with several pillows: one or two to support your elbow and hand on the side you'll be nursing on, one or two in your lap to bring the baby up to the level of your nipple, and perhaps one or two behind your back and shoulders for comfort and support. A footstool or something else on which to rest your feet is also helpful.

- You may want to pump your breasts before your baby's first feedings, especially if you have a forceful let-down reflex. Your baby can practice sucking without being overwhelmed by milk flow.

- Allow lots of time for early breastfeedings. Be calm and patient.

A nurse or lactation consultant may be available to assist you during these early feedings. The nurse may monitor your baby's condition and help you determine how much milk your baby has taken and when it is time to end the feeding. Having an extra pair of hands can be very helpful.

Correct positioning is important

Most pictures of breastfeeding mothers and babies show the baby's head resting in the bend of mother's elbow. This cradle-hold position does not work well for premies; they need a hand behind their heads for support. Try one of the following.

Cross-cradle hold. Place your baby on the pillows in your lap in a horizontal or semi-upright position. His mouth should be at the level of your nipple, with his whole body facing yours. If you are

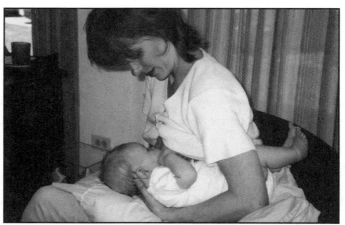

Top photo: football hold; bottom photo: cross cradle hold.

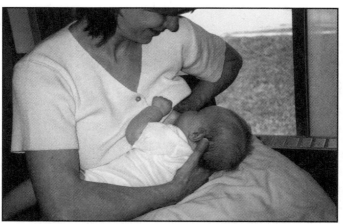

These positions are shown here with a larger baby; a premature baby may need some adjustments and more support.

breastfeeding on your left breast, place your right hand behind your baby's head to guide and support him, and use your left hand to support the breast. On the right side, you would use your left hand to support the baby's head and the right hand to offer the breast. Hold the breast with your thumb on top and fingers underneath, placed an inch or more behind the edge of the areola.

Football or clutch hold. If you are nursing on your left breast, your left hand supports the baby's head with his body at your side, tucked under your arm. Use a pillow or two under the baby and under your forearm to bring baby up to the level of the nipple.

Your right hand supports the breast. If you are nursing on the right breast, your right hand holds the baby and your left hand supports the breast.

If your baby's hands are active and making it difficult to achieve or maintain a correct breastfeeding position during the first few days, it may help to swaddle the baby snugly with his hands close to his body. Babies don't seem to mind this; it may even help the sleepy baby to awaken or the fussy baby to settle down.

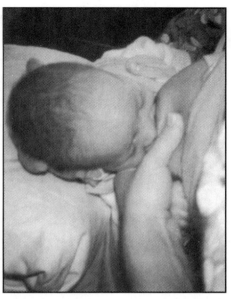

Supporting the breast with your hand helps baby stay latched on.

Getting the baby to latch on to the breast

Brush your nipple gently across the baby's lips. Express a few drops of milk to get him interested. You want him to open his mouth wide with his tongue down and flat. Some babies will do this right away. Others will make little sucking movements or will lick the nipple. When the baby does open his mouth wide, quickly pull him in closer to you, guiding his mouth onto the breast. Gentle pressure on the back of his head can help him stay on the breast.

The nipple and part of the areola should go way into the back of his mouth. If the baby takes only the nipple, remove him from the breast, calm him down if necessary, and try again. If the baby sucks only on the nipple, he will not get much milk and you will get very sore. Keep trying, and you and he will eventually get the technique working smoothly.

If your baby does not open his mouth, use the index finger of the hand supporting your breast to push down gently on his chin. (A nurse can help you with this at first, if you feel you need an extra hand.) Say "open" as you do this, and soon he will learn to associate the sound with the action. Then guide the breast into his mouth and quickly pull him in close to you.

How to tell if your baby is taking the breast properly. Getting the baby latched on correctly will prevent nipple soreness and enable the baby to suck effectively. Here are some points to check:

- The baby's lips should be flanged out and relaxed. Be sure he does not have his upper or lower lip drawn into his mouth along with your nipple.

- The baby's chin should touch your breast. The baby's nose may also touch your breast. The baby will still be able to breathe out the sides of his nose. Pressing down on the breast to make an airway usually is not necessary, and it can pull the nipple from the back of the baby's mouth to the front, making his sucking less effective.

- The lower jaw does most of the work in the sucking action. Be sure baby takes in a large portion of the lower part of the areola.

- The baby's tongue should be cupped under the breast. You can pull down gently on his lower lip to check this. If the tongue is not visible, take him off the breast and try again.

- The baby should not have to stretch or turn his head to reach your nipple.

- You should not have to bend over your baby with a tense neck and shoulders. Pull the baby toward you to get him close enough to reach your nipple; don't move your body toward him. Relax and let the pillows support you and him.

- A folded blanket or a small pillow can help support the hand behind the baby's head.

Premies may have trouble staying on the breast. Your hand should support the weight of the breast so that it doesn't rest on your baby's chin. You can hold your index finger under his chin to help him stay latched on. If he needs more support, use the Dancer hand position: slide the hand supporting the breast forward so that the thumb and the index finger form a U around the baby's jawline. The baby's chin rests in the bottom of the U and the thumb and finger help to support his jaw, while your other fingers support your breast. A nurse or another helper can maintain gentle pressure on the back of the baby's head to help him stay on the breast.

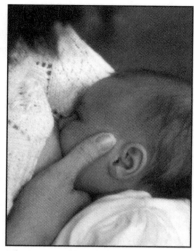

The Dancer Hand position provides extra support to keep baby latched on well.

Watch baby's sucking rhythm

After the baby has latched on, his first sucks will be rapid, small movements until the milk begins to flow. After the let-down reflex occurs, the sucking rhythm will change to deeper and slower sucks, and you will hear him swallow. This is a sure sign that he is getting milk. If he is sucking well, you will see a "wiggle" at his temple in front of his ears.

After a few minutes of rhythmic sucking, swallowing, and pausing, you will notice the sucking rhythm changing again, as the baby goes back to little sucks with swallows farther and farther apart and longer pauses. He may be ready to fall asleep at this point, and you may want to let him sleep. Since premies tire easily, he may be able to take only one breast during early feedings.

If he is still awake and alert, you can take him off the breast, burp him, and switch to the other side. If he has a good grasp of your breast, you will need to slide your finger into his mouth, between his gums, to release the suction. (Just "popping" a baby off the breast can make mother's nipples sore.) You can sit your baby in your lap to burp him, supporting his head and tummy with one hand and rubbing his back with the other. Or you can hold him up, with his tummy over your shoulder, and rub his back. He may or may not bring up air after a minute or two. After burping, switch the baby to the other side, and nurse him from the other breast until he drops off to sleep.

When to end a feeding

Don't limit your baby's time at the breast to a prescribed number of minutes. Instead, watch his signals to determine when he is tiring and needs to stop. A nurse can help you decide when your baby has had enough. Your baby may let you know that he's full or tired by ceasing to suck. Many babies fall asleep at the breast at the end of a feeding. Or your baby may show other signs of fatigue or stress.

During early feedings, your milk-ejection reflex may take longer to function, and the baby may suck for several minutes and fall asleep before your milk lets down. This can be frustrating, but it's perfectly normal. Your body will soon learn to respond to your baby's nursing, and your milk will let down sooner. Massaging or pumping your breasts for a few minutes before starting the feeding may stimulate the let-down reflex and bring the milk down sooner for your baby.

Remember that very tiny babies may not be able to tolerate switching from one breast to the other; movement, repositioning, and struggling to latch on tire them out, and they are then unable to nurse well. During early feedings your baby may be able to nurse only on one side. Watch his signals to avoid overtiring or stressing him. It's better for the baby to nurse well on only one breast than to nurse less effectively on both.

If the baby falls asleep early in the feeding you may be able to hold him skin-to-skin while he sleeps, and try again when he awakens. It's never a good idea to try to express milk into the mouth of a sleepy or tired newborn to encourage him to nurse; the unsuspecting baby may choke and aspirate the milk into his lungs.

Problems with Early Breastfeedings

If you and the baby are growing very frustrated with trying to nurse, take a break, calm the baby down, and relax for fifteen or twenty minutes before trying again. It may take several attempts—or even several sessions—to get your baby to latch on to the breast and suck. You may feel awkward at first, but don't blame yourself—it simply takes time.

The baby's first bursts of sucking will be short, but they will lengthen as he matures. It will take him a while to learn to suck steadily and to coordinate breathing and swallowing. As he approaches his original due date, his breastfeeding behavior will become more mature.

Don't worry about how much milk your baby is getting from the breast in these first nursing sessions. Focus on the learning process instead. With your patient support, your baby will begin to get the idea; he will latch on to the breast more readily and will suck for longer stretches.

If you experience sore nipples, pay close attention to the baby's position at the breast. Make sure he is taking some of the areola as well as the nipple into his mouth. You may need an extra pillow on your lap to keep the baby from slipping down off the areola and onto the nipple as he nurses. It shouldn't hurt to breastfeed. If you have sore nipples that aren't getting better, call a La Leche League Leader. She may have some more suggestions for you, or if not, she may be able to refer you to someone who has special training in working with sucking problems.

Measuring the Baby's Milk Intake

Physicians and neonatal nurses sometimes object to feeding premies at the breast because they think there is no way to know how much milk the baby has taken. Actually, there is a way to measure milk intake at the breast, a technique called test-weighing. The baby can be weighed before and after feedings, under identical conditions, on an electronic scale; the weight gain after the feeding, measured in grams, is equal to the amount of milk consumed, measured in milliliters. The baby should stay in the same clothes and the same diaper for both weighings, and the scale must be an electronic one. Mechanical scales are not accurate enough to detect the small increase in weight from the milk in baby's tummy.

Test-weighing can be very reassuring. Knowing how much milk the baby takes at the breast can help you and the doctors and nurses make decisions about your baby's care. It can be used to determine how much supplement the baby needs to receive. It can also help you recognize if your baby is breastfeeding effectively.

The results of test-weighing are not meant to be a judgment about your breastfeeding skills or your baby's. The amount of milk a baby takes at a feeding is just another piece of information that can be helpful in planning your baby's care. Sometimes your baby won't take very much milk at a feeding. This can be discouraging, but it can also prompt you to find new ways to encourage your baby to feed better. At other times, test-weighing will confirm your belief that your baby is nursing well.

Weighing may not be necessary during your baby's first feedings at the breast, when he is just learning to nurse and not taking much milk. But as time goes on, knowing how much milk your baby takes during breastfeeding will enable you and your baby's caregivers to ensure that he continues to gain weight as he makes the transition to getting all his nourishment at the breast. Eventually, as both you and your baby gain experience with breastfeeding, you will know that he is getting enough to eat by the number of wet and soiled diapers daily, by his breastfeeding behavior, and by his steady growth.

Supplementary Feedings

At first, your baby will be able to breastfeed for only one or two feedings a day. The other feedings of human milk or formula will be given by gavage or by bottle. Since artificial nipples require a different sucking action than the breast, bottles can cause problems. Some babies may become "nipple confused" when they receive supplemental feedings from bottles. This affects their feeding at the breast, making it more difficult to teach them to latch on and nurse. Ask your baby's care providers if it is possible for supplements to continue to be given by gavage at least during the first week that your baby is learning to breastfeed. Many nurseries are willing to do this, and it will make nursing easier for your baby.

Some hospitals may be willing to give supplementary feedings of human milk or formula using a cup, eyedropper, spoon, or feed-

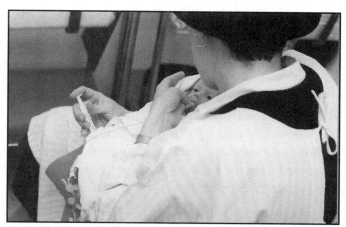

Finger-feeding: Mother uses a syringe to supply milk to her baby through tubing taped to her finger.

ing syringe. This is a way to avoid nipple confusion, but it does require extra effort from caregivers. Supplements can also be given while a baby is nursing at the breast, using a nursing supplementer. Another possibility is finger-feeding, using narrow tubing taped to a clean finger; as the baby sucks on the finger he gets milk through the tube, which is attached to a container of milk. Finger-feeding can also be done using a feeding syringe to supply milk while a baby sucks on a caregiver's finger. More information about how to use these alternatives to bottles can be found in Chapter 6.

There are many ways to give supplementary feedings to premies. How your baby will be fed when he is not nursing at the breast will depend on your preferences, his condition, and the willingness of your baby's caregivers to use these alternative feeding methods. Some of these alternatives to artificial nipples may be new to your baby's nurses. Remind them that avoiding artificial nipples can help your baby succeed at the breast. If you find that bottles are unavoidable, breastfeeding may require more patience on your part, but your baby will eventually master breastfeeding, especially if the baby is introduced to the breast before being offered a bottle. The more you can be at the hospital to breastfeed your baby, the fewer bottles he will get.

Continue pumping

You will need to continue pumping during the times when you can't be at the hospital for feedings. You may also want to pump at the hospital after feedings since your baby may not take much milk at first when he nurses. If you have been pumping for many weeks, your milk supply may be low at the point when your baby starts breastfeeding. At first, his nursing may not be vigorous or frequent enough to stimulate more milk production. Keep pumping at home and bringing the milk to the hospital for your baby to have when you can't be there.

When you are at the hospital, baby's feedings should be at the breast. Let the nurses know when you will be coming in each day—post a sign on the baby's isolette to remind them—so that you won't arrive to find that the baby has just been fed and is sound asleep. If possible, spend the entire day with your baby and feed him on demand at the hospital for a day or two before his homecoming. This can help boost your confidence as you learn to interpret his hunger cues.

Chapter 6
Coming Home

The day will finally arrive when it's time to take your baby home. You may have several days to prepare for this big event, or you may just get a phone call one morning from the hospital saying, "Today's the day." Either way, getting ready to take care of your baby full-time can be both joyful and worrisome. You're probably eager to feel like a "normal" family, and you want to start enjoying your baby. But you may also worry about your ability to care for this little one, especially if she continues to have special medical needs. Even after the doctors pronounce a little one healthy and growing well, the fears and difficulties of the past weeks tend to linger in parents' minds. Plus, adding a baby to your household demands big adjustments.

Baby's First Days at Home

Plan to spend your first days at home with your baby doing nothing but nursing, resting, and taking care of her needs. Get help with household tasks—the laundry, cleaning, cooking. Ask a friend or relative to come over and entertain your older children for several hours each day. Eat food from the freezer, ask helpful friends to bring meals, or order out. Now is a good time for fathers to take several days off from work, if possible, to spend time with the baby and to help take care of mother. Limit visitors, and ask those who do come to stay only a few minutes.

Getting enough sleep. The first weeks at home with your baby will be stressful. You'll need to eat well, drink plenty of fluids, and get enough rest; this will help you stay healthy and handle your worries better. Nap when your baby naps, at least once during the day.

Many mothers find that the easiest way to handle nighttime nursings is to bring the baby into bed with them. If your premie has difficulty nursing while you're lying down, you may want to move a big, comfortable chair, and maybe a footstool, into your room for nighttime nursings. Keep a blanket nearby to cover both of you. Or sit at the head of the bed with plenty of pillows behind your back, under your elbow, and at your side to support the baby at the breast. When the feeding is over, you can return the baby to her bed, or keep her next to you, so you won't have to get out of bed for the next feeding.

Tiny babies love to sleep on their parents' chests; they hear the heartbeat and sense the regular breathing rhythm and feel right at home. A bed rail, like those made for toddlers who are learning to sleep in a big bed, can guard against falls. Or push the bed up against the wall. (For more on sharing sleep with your baby see NIGHTTIME PARENTING by William Sears, available from bookstores and LLLI.)

Breastfeeding at Home

Feeding your baby is likely to be high on your list of concerns. Worries about whether the baby is getting enough milk are very common among breastfeeding mothers of premies—and mothers of breastfed full-term infants, too. Learning to trust a natural process such as breastfeeding can be difficult in a society that has become accustomed to technological solutions. And while breastfeeding is nature's superior way of nourishing infants, it doesn't necessarily come naturally. Your first weeks of breastfeeding your baby at home will be a learning experience.

Many mothers find that they need lots of emotional support in these early weeks of caring for their babies. Call a La Leche League Leader if you want to talk things over with someone who has a positive attitude toward breastfeeding. You may also be able to call a lactation specialist at the hospital for suggestions or just a listening ear. Friends who have breastfed their babies may also be able to give you encouragement, though they may not understand the special challenges of nursing a baby who has spent her early weeks in the hospital.

Your milk supply. Your body can produce enough milk for your growing baby. It is very rare for a woman not to be able to make enough milk for one baby, or even two. Delivering prematurely does not affect milk-making abilities. However, when a baby takes very little milk at the breast in each feeding a mother's milk supply may dwindle. And a baby who is not yet an efficient nurser is not able to build up a mother's milk supply the way a more experienced nursing baby can. This is why it is important to keep pumping after feedings until your baby learns to nurse well and can get most of her nourishment at the breast.

Pumping will provide milk that can be given to your baby as a supplement. It will also increase your milk supply and increase the amount of milk released when you have a let-down. Having more milk than your baby actually needs means your baby won't have to work as hard to get the milk from your breasts. This can be important to babies who have not yet perfected their sucking technique.

How to Tell If Baby Is Getting Enough Milk

There are different approaches to monitoring a premature baby's human milk intake and growth in the weeks after leaving the hospital. What works best for you and your baby will depend on how well your baby is nursing, her size and maturity, the preferences of the baby's doctor, your own worries and concerns, and other related factors.

The electronic scale. One approach is to monitor the baby's milk intake with an electronic scale, as is done in many hospitals.

Electronic scales can be rented for use at home after your baby is discharged. (See Resources.) With a note from your physician, your insurance company should pay for this.

Being able to measure how much milk the baby takes at every feeding helps many mothers feel more confident that their premie is getting enough to eat. They use the information on milk intake at the breast to determine exactly how much supplement to give the baby from day to day. Because they don't have to wonder whether baby is getting enough milk, they may find it easier to make the transition to exclusive breastfeeding.

Dr. Paula Meier, a neonatal nurse and researcher who has studied the test-weighing technique in premature infants, suggests the following approach to giving supplements. The baby's doctor determines how much milk the baby needs in 24 hours, and from this determines how much milk the baby should get in each six- or eight-hour period through the day. The mother can then watch her baby's cues and feed her on demand, while keeping track of how much the baby takes at each feeding. Every six or eight hours the mother adds up these amounts, subtracts the total from the amount of milk the baby should get every six or eight hours, and then gives the baby the necessary amount of supplement (human milk or formula) to make up the difference. This plan makes it possible to offer supplementary feedings just three or four times a day, instead of after every breastfeeding.

Eventually a mother who is weighing her baby before and after feedings will rely on other ways to recognize that the baby is truly getting enough milk at the breast. She will know from experience when the baby has nursed well. As the baby becomes better at breastfeeding, the mother can switch to weighing the baby only once a day, and then every two or three days, to be certain she is continuing to grow. After a few weeks, frequent weight checks will no longer be necessary.

Other ways to tell if the baby is nursing well

Here are some clues from the baby's behavior that can help you know if your baby is getting enough to eat:

- Your baby is swallowing after every one or two sucks for five to ten minutes on each side at every feeding.

- Your baby is nursing eight or more times in twenty-four hours.

- Your baby has six to eight wet diapers every day and, most important, two to five bowel movements daily. If she has only two bowel movements, the amount should be substantial. More frequent bowel movements may be little more than a stain on the diaper after every feeding. (An older breastfed baby may go several days between bowel movements. This does not mean the baby is constipated unless stools are hard and dry.)

- If your baby has been getting formula supplements, you will notice that her stool changes as she gets more and more of your milk. The breastfed baby's stool is soft and yellow to tan in color, with only a mild odor.

Giving supplements

Usually, it's best to feed the baby at the breast before offering supplements of human milk or formula. You may want to give the supplement by spoon, eyedropper, feeding syringe, or cup in order to avoid using artificial nipples, especially if your baby has been having trouble learning to nurse at the breast. However, many premies do learn to take both the breast and a bottle nipple.

The idea of cup-feeding a little baby may seem strange at first, but babies actually learn to sip from a cup surprisingly easily. Follow these steps to cup-feed your baby:

- Choose a small clean cup or glass. A flexible plastic cup about the size of a shot glass works well.

- Fill the cup at least half full.

- Be sure the baby is awake and alert.

- Swaddle the baby in a blanket to keep her hands from bumping the cup. Use a bib or a cloth diaper under her chin in case of spills.

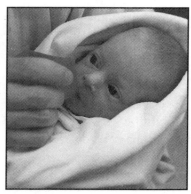

Cup feeding

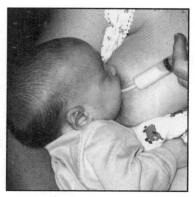

Finger feeding with a syringe and tubing

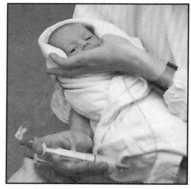

Using a feeding syringe at the breast

- Hold the baby on your lap in an upright position.

- Bring the cup to the baby's lips, gently tilting it so that when she opens her mouth the cup rests lightly on her lower lip and the milk just touches her lips.

- Tip the cup slightly so that a few drops of milk flow onto the baby's lips, but do not put milk in the baby's mouth.

- Leave the cup in this position and let the baby set her own sipping rhythm. Let her pause when needed, and end the feeding when she is tired.

Another option is to use a nursing supplementer, a device that makes it possible for the baby to receive supplementary milk while nursing at the breast. A tiny tube extends from a bottle to the mother's nipple; when the baby nurses, she gets milk from the bottle as well as from the breast. The height of the bottle and the size of the tubing determine how fast the milk flows. Some mothers dislike having to use devices while nursing their babies; others prefer using the supplementer because it keeps the baby at the breast. Some mothers start to use the supplementer while their baby is still in the hospital. A nursing supplementer can also be used for finger-feeding by taping the tube to a clean finger. Your La Leche League Leader can tell you where you can purchase a supplementer and help you learn how to use it. You can also buy special devices designed especially for finger-feeding.

Keep a notebook or a chart that shows how often your baby nurses each day, how much supplement she takes, and the number of wet diapers and bowel movements. As the days go by, you will see the amount of supplement she takes decrease, an indication that your baby is getting more milk at the breast. How quickly a baby goes from nursing-and-supplementing to exclusive breastfeeding varies a great deal, but keeping daily records for a while will help you become confident that your baby is doing well at the breast.

The doctor will monitor your baby's growth closely in the weeks after she leaves the hospital. You will probably find that weight checks are very reassuring, and that your baby is growing well on mother's milk.

Establishing a feeding routine

During your first week or two at home with your baby, it may seem as if feeding takes up most of your waking hours. By the time you feed the baby at the breast, weigh her before and after the feeding, write down the results, prepare and offer the supplement, burp the baby, and pump your breasts to stimulate your milk supply, it may be time to start all over again. Breastfeeding may feel like a huge commitment at this point, and family and friends may wonder why you are going to all this trouble. It helps to remember that 1) your baby benefits enormously from receiving your milk, and 2) breastfeeding will get easier—and even save you time in the long run. One way to save time right now is to have dad or a helper give baby the supplement while you pump. Some mothers also manage to pump one breast while baby is nursing at the other.

Breastfeeding on cue. In the hospital, your baby may have been fed every three or four hours by the clock, because that was the hospital routine. But babies don't read clocks. At home, you'll want to follow your baby's cues and feed her whenever she seems to need to nurse. Babies breastfeed very frequently in the early months, but those feedings are not usually evenly spaced over twenty-four hours. Sometimes your baby may want to nurse again an hour or less after the last feeding. Once or twice a day she may go three or four hours between feedings. This is perfectly normal. Remember that babies nurse for comfort as well as for food.

If your baby is nursing fewer than eight times a day, you should encourage her to nurse more frequently. Premies do need more sleep than full-term babies, but if your baby is sleeping long stretches during the day (more than two or three hours), watch for times when she is mouthing and moving about in her sleep; this is a good time to pick her up and encourage her to nurse. Besides getting more milk into her, this may also encourage your baby to take her long naps at night.

A Time of Adjustment

Premies are more sensitive than full-term babies. They are easily overwhelmed by the stimulation in their environment, and all the time spent in the hustle and bustle and noise of the neonatal intensive care nursery does not help them learn to calm down. Breastfeeding, with its rhythmic sucking, the warmth of being close to mother, the comfort of warm, sweet milk, will help your baby learn to trust you and have confidence in herself. You may find that when your baby has been fussy, she nurses better in a quiet, dimly lit place. Even talking to her may disturb her while she is busy at the breast.

Give your baby lots of peaceful holding, rocking, and body contact for much of the day. Use a baby carrier to keep her with you around the house and when you go out. A sling-type carrier may be more adaptable to her size and needs than a front-pack carrier. (Use a folded blanket in the bottom of the sling for extra support if your baby seems to get lost in the fabric.) Remember that responding to your baby's cries and whimpers will not spoil her; it will help her learn to trust you and herself. Crying is not good for babies. This is especially true for premies. For more tips on soothing and mothering your baby, see THE FUSSY BABY by William Sears and THE WOMANLY ART OF BREASTFEEDING.

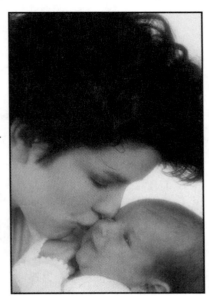

The experience of premature labor and birth, followed by weeks of worry about a baby in the hospital, is a difficult one, and it may be many months before you feel like a "normal" family. But as your baby grows, develops, and reveals her own individual personality, she will cease to be your "premie" and will become simply herself. Meanwhile, you will gain confidence in your own ability to mother your child and to understand her.

The outlook for premature infants is better than ever. Breastfeeding can be a way for you and your baby to know and enjoy one another and for you to gain confidence in yourself as a mother. You'll know that you're giving your precious child the very best in nutrition, along with lots of love.

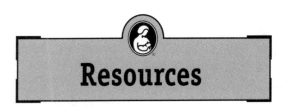

Resources

Publications

Davis, D. L. *Empty Cradle, Broken Heart*. Golden, CO: Fulcrum, 1991. A guide for parents whose baby dies.

Gotsch, Gwen. BREASTFEEDING PURE AND SIMPLE. La Leche League International, 1993. A clear, concise introduction to breastfeeding.

La Leche League International. THE WOMANLY ART OF BREASTFEEDING, 6th ed. La Leche League International, 1997. La Leche League's basic manual covering all aspects of breastfeeding.

Ludington-Hoe, S. M. and Golant, S. K. *Kangaroo Care: The Best You Can Do to Help Your Preterm Infant*. New York: Bantam, 1993.

Popper, Barbara. *The Hospitalized Nursing Baby—Meeting the Needs of Mothers, Babies, and Families in Health Care Settings*. La Leche League International, 1998. Tells how breastfeeding can and should be protected and continued when either the mother or baby is hospitalized.

Sears, William. THE FUSSY BABY: *How to Bring Out the Best in Your High Need Child*. La Leche League International, 1985. Written by a pediatrician and father, this book offers support and reassurance as well as practical tips for parents of "high-need" babies.

Sears, William. NIGHTTIME PARENTING: *How to Get Your Baby and Child to Sleep*. La Leche League International, 1985. Explains the differences in babies' sleeping patterns compared to those of adults and discusses sleep-sharing as a style of nighttime parenting.

Sears, William. *SIDS: A Parent's Guide to Understanding and Preventing Sudden Infant Death Syndrome*. Little, Brown and Company, 1995. A comprehensive review of research on Sudden Infant Death Syndrome with suggestions on minimizing the risks.

Zaichkin, Jeanette. *Newborn Intensive Care: What Every Parent Needs to Know*. Petaluma, CA: NICU Ink, 1996. Comprehensive information on the health challenges faced by premature infants and the technology used to care for them. (Available from Childbirth Graphics, 800-299-3366, ext. 287; fax 888-977-7653, $24.95.)

La Leche League International

La Leche League International provides information, encouragement, and mother-to-mother support to mothers who want to breastfeed their babies. A network of volunteer Leaders hold meetings and answer questions by phone in communities across the United States, Canada, and other countries worldwide. To obtain the name of a Leader near you, call 1-800-LA-LECHE (in the USA), 1-800-665-4324 (in Canada) or 1-847-519-7730. You can also send a fax to 1-847-519-0035 or an email to lllhq@llli.org. You can also visit the La Leche League International Website at www.lalecheleague.org.

Most of the books listed above are available through the LLLI Catalogue, along with breast pumps, feeding devices, and milk storage systems. You can request a free copy by calling the numbers listed above or writing to LLLI, PO Box 4079, Schaumburg, IL 60168-4079 USA or, in Canada, write to LLL Canada, 18-C Industrial Drive, Chesterville K0C1H0 Canada.

Pumps, Electronic Scales, and Feeding Devices

To find information on buying or renting breast pumps, electronic scales, and supplementary feeding devices, contact:

Medela	**Hollister Incorporated**
P.O. Box 660	2000 Hollister Drive
McHenry, IL 60051-0660 USA	Libertyville, IL 60048 USA
Telephone: 1-800-435-8316	Telephone: 1-800-323-4060
Website: www.medela.com	Canada: 1-800-263-7400

Lansinoh for Breastfeeding Mothers®

Created especially for nursing mothers who need relief from sore nipples. Using a patented process that removes allergens and impurities, Lansinoh is the world's purest lanolin. Lansinoh does not have to be removed prior to nursing and can be used with complete confidence of safety for mother and baby. You can purchase Lansinoh from LLLI. No. 581: 2 oz. for $9.95 and No. 582: 1/4 oz. for $2.50. Also available in many drugstores and discount stores.

Donor Milk Banks

For information on storing human milk and donor milk banks please contact:

The Human Milk Banking Association of North America
P.O. Box 370464
West Hartford, CT 06137-0464
Website: www.leron-line.com/milkbank.htm

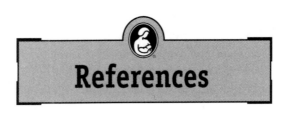

References

This bibliography will be useful to health care professionals and others interested in the research this book is based on. The references are organized by topics that correspond to sections in this book. Sharing this information with your baby's caregivers can help them be more supportive of your efforts to breastfeed your baby.

General Background

Hill, P. et al. Mothers of low birthweight infants: breastfeeding patterns and problems. *J Hum Lact* 1994; 10(3):169-76.

Kavanaugh, K. L., Meier, P., Zimmerman, B., and Mead, L. P. The rewards outweigh the efforts: Breastfeeding outcomes for mothers of preterm infants. *J Hum Lact* 1997; 13:15-21.

McCoy, R., Kadowaki, C., Wilks, S., Engstrom, J., and Meier, P. Nursing management of breast feeding for preterm infants. *J Perinat Neonatal Nurs* 1988; 2(1):42-55.

Meier, P., Brown, L. P., and Hurst, N. M. Breastfeeding the pre-term infant. In *Breastfeeding and Human Lactation 2nd Edition,* eds. J. Riordan and K. Auerbach, 449-481. Sudbury, MA: Jones and Bartlett, 1999.

Mohrbacher, N. and Stock, J. THE BREASTFEEDING ANSWER BOOK, rev. ed. Schaumburg, IL: La Leche League International, 1997.

Walker, M. Breastfeeding the premature infant. *NAACOG Clin Issues Perinat Women Health Nurs* 1992; 3(4):620-33.

Walker, M. BREASTFEEDING PREMATURE BABIES. Unit 14. La Leche League International Lactation Consultant Series. Garden City Park, New York: Avery, 1990.

Why human milk is important for premature infants

American Academy of Pediatrics Work Group on Breastfeeding. Breastfeeding and the use of human milk. *Pediatrics* 1997; 100:1035-39.

Buescher, E. S. Host defense mechanisms of human milk and their relations to enteric infections and necrotizing enterocolitis. *Clin Perinatol* 1994; 21(2):247-62.

Clandinin, M. et al. Requirements of newborn infants for long chain polyunsaturated fatty acids. *Acta Paediatr Scand* Suppl 1989; 351:63-71.

deCurtis, M., Paone, C., Betrono, G. et al. A case control study of necrotizing enterocolitis occurring over 8 years in a neonatal intensive care unit. *Eur J Pediatr* 1979; 146:450.

Gale, S. et al. Is dietary epidermal growth factor absorbed by premature human infants? *Biol Neonate* 1989; 55:104-10.

Hamosh, M. Digestion in the premature infant: The effects of human milk. *Sem Perinatol* 1994; 18:485-94.

Lucas, A. and Cole, T. Breast milk and neonatal necrotizing enterocolitis. *Lancet* 1990; 336:1519.

Lucas, A. et al. Breast milk and subsequent intelligence quotient in children born preterm. *Lancet* 1992; 339:261-64.

Luukkainen, P. et al. Changes in the fatty acid composition of preterm and term human milk from 1 week to 6 months of lactation. *J Pediatr Gastroenterol Nutr* 1994; 18:355-60.

Nutrition Committee Canadian Paediatric Society. Nutrient needs and feeding of premature infants. *Can Med Assoc J* 1995; 152(11):1765-85.

Parsa, N. et al. Role of breastfeeding in necrotizing enterocolitis in preterm infants. *Am J Epidemiol* 1994; 139(11):S73.

Rogan, W. and Gladen, B. Breastfeeding and cognitive development. *Early Human Dev* 1993; 31:181-93.

Schanler, R. and Hurst, N. Human milk for the hospitalized preterm infant. *Sem Perinatol* 1994; 18(6):476-84.

Uauy, R. et al. Effect of dietary omega-3 fatty acids in retinal function of very-low-birth-weight neonates. *Pediatr Res* 1990; 28:485-92.

Expressing and storing human milk

Auerbach, K. Sequential and simultaneous breast pumping: a comparison. *Int J Nurs Stud* 1990; 27(3):257-65.

deCarvalho, M. et al. Frequency of milk expression and milk production by mothers of non-nursing premature neonates. *Am J Dis Child* 1985; 139:483-87.

Hamosh, M., Ellis, L. A., Pollock, D. R. et al. Breastfeeding and the working mother: Effect of time and temperature of short-term storage on proteolysis, lipolysis, and bacterial growth in milk. *Pediatrics* 1996; 97:492-98.

Hill, P. D., Brown, L. P., and Harker, T. L. Initiation and frequency of breast expression in breastfeeding mothers of LBW and VLBW infants. *Nurs Res* 1995; 44:352-55.

Hill, P. D., Aldag, J. C., and Chatterton, R. T. The effect of sequential and simultaneous breast pumping on milk volume and prolactin levels: A pilot study. *J Hum Lact* 1996; 12:193-99.

The Human Milk Banking Association of North America. *Recommendations for Collection, Storage, and Handling of a Mother's Milk for Her Own Infant in the Hospital Setting.* West Hartford, CT, 1993.

Law, B. J., Urias, B. A., Lertzman, J. et al. Is ingestion of milk-associated bacteria by preterm infants fed raw human milk controlled by routine bacteriologic screening? *J Clin Microbiol* 1989; 27: 1560-66.

Mohrbacher, N. and Stock, J. THE BREASTFEEDING ANSWER BOOK, rev. ed. Schaumburg, IL: La Leche League International, 1997.

Schanler, R. and Hurst, N. Human milk for the hospitalized preterm infant. *Sem Perinatol* 1994; 18(6):476-84.

Tube-feeding of human milk and human milk fortification

Bishop, N. et al. Early diet of preterm infants and bone mineralization at age five years. *Acta Paediatr* 1996; 85:230-36.

Brennan-Behm, M., Carlson, E., Meier, P. et al. Caloric loss from expressed mother's milk during continuous gavage infusions of breast milk. *Neonatal Network* 1994; 13:27-32.

Brook, O. G. and Barley, J. Loss of energy during continuous infusions of breast milk. *Arch Dis Child* 1978; 53:344-45.

Greer, F., McCormick, A., and Loker, J. Changes in fat concentration of human milk during delivery by intermittent bolus and continuous mechanical pump infusion. *J Pediatr* 1984; 105:745.

Jarvenpaa, A. et al. Preterm infants fed human milk attain intrauterine weight gain. *Acta Paediatr Scand* 1983; 72:239-43.

Lucas, A., Fewtrell, M. S., Morley, R. et al. Randomized outcome trial of human milk fortification and developmental outcome in preterm infants. *Am J Clin Nutr* 1996; 64:142-51.

Schanler, R. Suitability of human milk for the low-birthweight infant. *Clin Perinatol* 1995; 22(1):207-22.

Schanler, R. and Abrams, S. Postnatal attainment of intrauterine macromineral accretion rates in low birth weight infants fed fortified human milk. *J Pediatr* 1995; 126:441-47.

Schanler, R. et al. Bone mineralization outcomes in human milk-fed preterm infants. *Pediatr Res* 1992; 31(6):583-86.

Valentine, C. et al. Hindmilk improves weight gain in low birthweight infants fed human milk. *J Pediatr Gastroenterol Nutr* 1994; 18:474-77.

Medications in human milk

American Academy of Pediatrics Committee on Drugs. The transfer of drugs and other chemicals into human milk. *Pediatrics* 1994; 93:137-50. Reprinted in THE BREASTFEEDING ANSWER BOOK, rev. ed. by N. Mohrbacher and J. Stock. Schaumburg, IL: La Leche League International, 1997, 525-538.

Briggs, G., Freeman, R., and Yaffe, S. *Drugs in Pregnancy and Lactation,* 5th ed. Baltimore: Williams and Wilkins, 1998.

Hale, T. *Medications and Mother's Milk,* 7th ed. Amarillo, TX: Pharmasoft, 1998-99. Also see Dr. Hale's website at http://neonatal.ttuhsc.edu/lact/index.html

Lawrence, R. *Breastfeeding: A Guide for the Medical Profession,* 5th ed. St. Louis: Mosby, 1999.

Kangaroo care

Acolet, D., K. Sleath, and A. Whitelaw. Oxygenation, heart rate and temperature in very low birthweight infants during skin-to-skin contact with their mothers. *Acta Paediatr Scand* 1989; 78:189-93.

Affonso, D. D., V. Wahlberg, and B. Persson. Exploration of mothers' reactions to the kangaroo method of prematurity care. *Neonatal Network* 1989; 7:43-51.

Als, H. et al. Individualized developmental care for the very low birth weight preterm infant: medical and neurofunctional effects. *JAMA* 1994; 272(11):853-58.

Anderson, G. C. Kangaroo care and breastfeeding for preterm infants. BREASTFEEDING ABSTRACTS 1989; 9:7-8.

Anderson, G. C. Current knowledge about skin-to-skin (Kangaroo) care for preterm infants. *J Perinatol* 1991; 11:216-26.

De Leeuw, R., Colin, E. M., Dunnebier, E. A., and Mirmiran, M. Physiological effects of kangaroo care in very small preterm infants. *Biol Neonate* 1991; 59:149-55.

Gale, G., Franck, L., and Lund, C. Skin-to-skin (Kangaroo) holding of the intubated premature infant. *Neonatal Network* 1993; 12:49-57.

Hadeed, A. et al. Skin to skin contact (SSC) between mother and infants reduces idiopathic apnea of prematurity (IAOP). *Pediatr Res* 1995; 37(4, pt 2):1233.

Hurst, N. M., Valentine, C. J., Renfro, L. et al. Skin-to-skin holding in the neonatal intensive care unit influences maternal milk volume. *J Perinatol* 1997; 17:213-17.

Karlsson, H. Skin-to-skin care: Heat balance. *Arch Dis Child* 1996; 75:F130-32.

Ludington-Hoe, S. M. Energy conservation during Kangaroo Care. *Heart and Lung* 1990; 19:445-51.

Ludington-Hoe, S. M. and Golant, S. K. *Kangaroo Care: The Best You Can Do to Help Your Preterm Infant.* New York: Bantam, 1993.

Ludington-Hoe, S. M., Hadeed, A., and Anderson, G. C. Physiologic responses to skin-to-skin contact in hospitalized premature infants. *J Perinatol* 1991; 11:19-24.

Sloan, N. et al. Kangaroo mother method: randomised controlled trial of an alternative method of care for stabilised low-birthweight infants. *Lancet* 1994; 344:182-85.

Feeding premature infants at the breast

Meier, P. Bottle and breast feeding: Effects on transcutaneous oxygen pressure and temperature in small preterm infants. *Nurs Res* 1988: 37:36-41.

Meier, P. and Anderson, G. Responses of preterm infants to bottle and breast feeding. *MCN* 1987; 12:97-105.

Meier, P., McCoy, R., and Mangurten, H. H. Management of breastfeeding for preterm infants. BREASTFEEDING ABSTRACTS 1988; 8:1-2.

Meier, P. and Pugh, E. J. Breast-feeding behavior of small preterm infants. *MCN* 1985; 10:396-400.

Avoiding bottles for supplementary feedings

Lang, S. et al. Cup feeding: An alternative method of infant feeding. *Arch Dis Child* 1994; 71:365-69.

Newman, J. Breastfeeding and problems associated with early introduction of bottles and pacifiers. *J Hum Lact* 1990; 6(2):59-63.

Stine, M. Breastfeeding the premature newborn: a protocol without bottles. *J Hum Lact* 1990; 6(4):167-70.

Test-weighing

Meier, P. et al. The accuracy of test weighing for preterm infants. *J Pediar Gastroenterol Nutr* 1990; 5:50-52.

Kavanaugh, K. et al. Getting enough: Mothers' concerns about breastfeeding a premature infant after discharge. *JOGN Nurs* 1995; 24(1):23-32.

Index